The Super Easy KETO Chaffle Cooking Guide For Beginners

Simple And Tasty Keto Chaffle Recipes

Lily Sherman

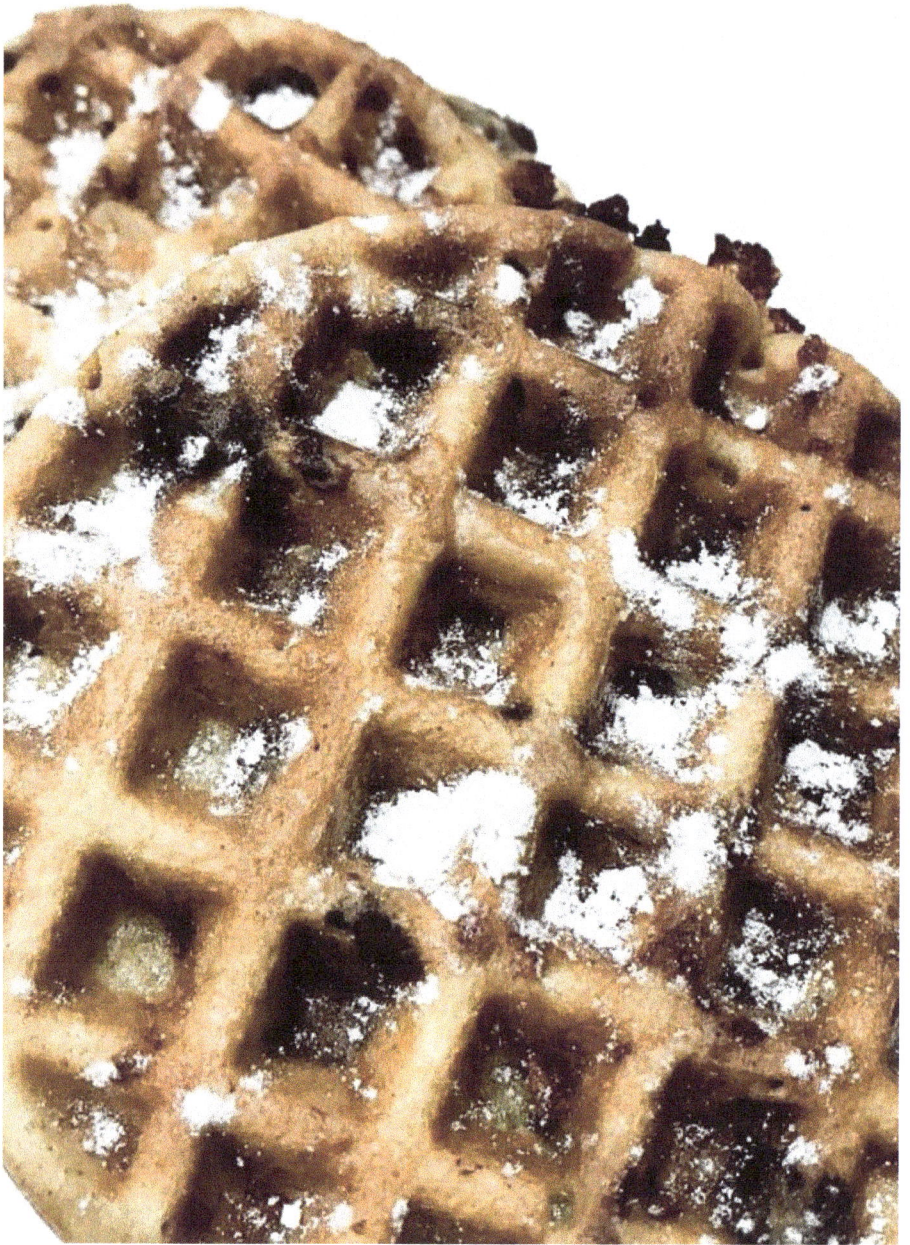

Table of contents

Chaffle Cannoli

Cooking: 28 Minutes

Servings: 4

Ingredients

For the chaffles:

- 1 large egg
- 1 egg yolk
- 3 tbsp butter, Melted
- 1 tbsp swerve confectioner's
- 1 cup finely grated Parmesan cheese
- 2 tbsp finely grated mozzarella cheese

For the cannoli filling:

- ½ cup ricotta cheese
- 2 tbsp swerve confectioner's sugar
- 1 tsp vanilla extract
- 2 tbsp unsweetened chocolate chips for garnishing

Directions

1. Preheat now the waffle iron.

2. Meanwhile, in a bowl, mix all the Ingredients for the chaffles.

3. Open the iron, pour in a quarter of the mixture, cover, and cook until crispy, 7 minutes.

4. Remove now the chaffle onto a plate and make 3 more with the remaining batter.

5. Meanwhile, for the cannoli filling:

6. Beat the ricotta cheese and swerve confectioner's sugar until smooth. Mix in the vanilla.

7. On each chaffle, spread some of the filling and wrap over.

8. Garnish the creamy ends with some chocolate chips.

9. Serve immediately.

Nutrition:

Calories 308, Fats 25.05g, Carbs 5.17g, Net Carbs 5.17g, Protein 15.18g

Blueberry Cream Cheese Chaffles

Cooking: 8 Minutes

Servings: 2

Ingredients

- 1 organic egg, beaten
- 1 tbspn cream cheese, softened
- 3 tbsps almond flour
- ¼ teaspn organic baking powder
- 1 teaspn organic blueberry extract
- 5-6 fresh blueberries

Directions

- Preheat now a mini waffle iron and then grease it.
- Place all the Ingredients except blueberries and beat until well combined in a bowl.
- Fold in the blueberries.
- Divide the mixture into 5 portions.
- Place 1 portion of the mixture into Preheated waffle iron and cook for about 3-4 minutes or until golden brown.

- Repeat now with the remaining mixture.
- Serve warm.

Nutrition:

Calories: 120, Fat: 9.6g, Saturated Fat: 2.2g, Carbohydrates: 3.1g, Dietary Fiber: 1.3g, Sugar: 1g, Protein: 3.2g

Italian Cream Chaffle Sandwich-cake

Cooking: 20 Minutes

Servings: 4

Ingredients

- 4 oz cream cheese, softened, at room temperature
- 4 eggs
- 1 Tbsp Melted butter
- 1 tsp vanilla extract
- ½ tsp cinnamon
- 1 Tbsp monk fruit sweetener
- 4 Tbsp coconut flour
- 1 Tbsp almond flour
- 1½ teaspns baking powder
- 1 Tbsp coconut, shredded and unsweetened
- 1 Tbsp walnuts, chopped

For the Italian cream frosting:

- 2 oz cream cheese, softened, at room temperature
- 2 Tbsp butter room temp
- 2 Tbsp monk fruit sweetener
- ½ tsp vanilla

Directions

1. Combine cream cheese, eggs, melted butter, vanilla, sweetener, flours, and baking powder in a blender.
2. Add walnuts and coconut to the mixture.
3. Blend to get a creamy mixture.
4. Turn on waffle maker to heat and oil it with cooking spray.
5. Add enough batter to fill waffle maker. Cook for 2-3 min, until chaffles are done.
6. Remove now and let them cool.
7. Mix all frosting Ingredients in another bowl. Stir until smooth and creamy.
8. Frost the chaffles once they have cooled.
9. Top with cream and more nuts.

Nutrition:

Carbs: 31 g, Fat: 2 g, Protein: 5 g, Calories: 168

Whipping Cream Chaffles

Cooking: 8 Minutes

Servings: 2

Ingredients

- 1 organic egg, beaten
- 1 tbspn heavy whipping cream
- 2 tbsps sugar-free peanut butter powder
- 2 tbsps Erythritol
- ¼ teaspn organic baking powder
- ¼ teaspn peanut butter extract

Directions

- Preheat now a mini waffle iron and then grease it.
- In a bowl, place all Ingredients and with a fork, mix well until well combined.
- Place half of the mixture into preheated waffle iron and cook for about 4 minutes or until golden brown.
- Repeat now with the remaining mixture.
- Serve warm.

Nutrition:

Calories: 112, Net Carb: 1g, Fat: 6.9g, Saturated Fat: 2.7g, Carbohydrates: 3.7g, Dietary Fiber: 2.1g, Sugar: 0.2g, Protein: 10.9g

Cinnamon Pumpkin Chaffles

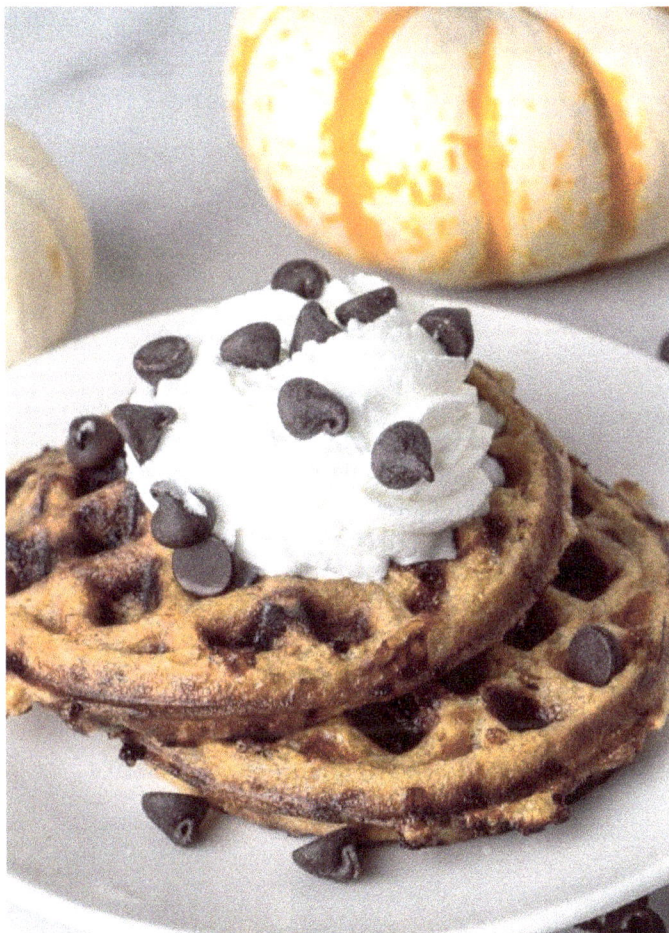

Cooking: 16 Minutes

Servings: 4

Ingredients

- 2 organic eggs
- 2/3 cup Mozzarella cheese, shredded
- 3 tbsps sugar-free pumpkin puree
- 3 teaspns almond flour
- 2 teaspns granulated Erythritol
- 2 teaspns ground cinnamon

Directions

- Preheat now a mini waffle iron and then grease it.
- In a bowl, place all Ingredients and with a fork, Mix well until well combined.
- Place half of the mixture into preheated waffle iron and cook for about 4 minutes or until golden brown.
- Repeat now with the remaining mixture.
- Serve warm.

Nutrition:

Net Carb: 1.4g, Fat: 4g, Saturated Fat: 1.3g, Carbohydrates: 2.5g, Dietary Fiber: 1.1g, Sugar: 0.6g, Protein: 4.3g

Strawberry cake Chaffles

Preparation: 5 minutes

Cooking: 25 Minutes

Servings: 1

Ingredients

For the Batter:

- 1 egg
- ¼ cup mozzarella cheese
- 1 Tbsp cream cheese
- ¼ tsp baking powder
- 2 strawberries, sliced
- 1 tsp strawberry extract

For the glaze:

- 1 Tbsp cream cheese
- ¼ tsp strawberry extract
- 1 Tbsp monk fruit confectioner's blend

For the whipped cream:

- 1 cup heavy whipping cream
- 1 tsp vanilla

- 1 Tbsp monk fruit

Directions

1. Turn on waffle maker to heat and oil it with cooking spray.
2. Beat egg in a tiny bowl.
3. Add remaining batter components.
4. Divide the mixture in half.
5. Cook one half of the batter in a waffle maker for 4 min, or until golden brown.
6. Repeat now with remaining batter
7. Mix all glaze Ingredients and spread over each warm chaffle.
8. Mix all whipped cream Ingredients and whip until it starts to form peaks.
9. Top each waffle with whipped cream and strawberries.

Nutrition:

Calories: 213, Fat: 10g, Protein: 9g, Carbohydrates: 20g, Fiber: 15g

Cream Cheese & Butter Chaffle

Preparation: 8 minutes

Cooking: 16 Minutes

Servings: 2

Ingredients

- 2 tbsps butter, melted and cooled
- 2 large organic eggs
- 2 ounce ofs cream cheese, softened
- ¼ cup powdered Erythritol
- 1½ teaspns organic vanilla extract
- Pinch of salt
- ¼ cup almond flour
- 2 tbsps coconut flour
- 1 teaspn organic baking powder

Directions

- Preheat now a mini waffle iron and then grease it.
- In a bowl, place the butter and eggs and beat until creamy.

- Add cream cheese, Erythritol, vanilla extract, salt, and beat until well combined.
- Add the flours and baking powder and beat until well combined.
- Place ¼ of the mixture into preheated waffle iron and cook for about 4 minutes or until golden brown.
- Repeat now with the remaining mixture.
- Serve warm.

Nutrition:

Calories: 230, Fat: 5g, Protein: 7g, Carbohydrates: 40g

Coconut and Walnut Chaffles

Preparation: 5 minutes

Cooking: 24 Minutes

Servings: 8

Ingredients

- 4 organic eggs, beaten
- 4 ounce ofs cream cheese, softened
- 1 tbspn butter, Melted
- 4 tbsps coconut flour
- 1 tbspn almond flour
- 2 tbsps Erythritol
- 1½ teaspns organic baking powder
- 1 teaspn organic vanilla extract
- ½ teaspn ground cinnamon
- 1 tbspn unsweetened coconut, shredded
- 1 tbspn walnuts, chopped

Directions

- Preheat now a mini waffle iron and then grease it.

- In a blender, place all Ingredients and pulse until creamy and smooth.
- Divide the mixture into 8 portions.
- Place 1 portion of the mixture into preheated waffle iron and cook for about 2-3 minutes or until golden brown.
- Repeat now with the remaining mixture.
- Serve warm.

Nutrition:

Calories: 289, Fat: 8g, Protein: 9g, Carbohydrates: 52g, Fiber: 10g

Chocolate cheese Chaffles

Preparation: 8 minutes

Cooking: 8 Minutes

Servings: 2

Ingredients

- 2 organic eggs
- ½ cup Mozzarella cheese, shredded
- ¾ teaspn organic lemon extract
- ½ teaspn organic vanilla extract
- 2 teaspns Erythritol
- ½ teaspn psyllium husk powder
- Pinch of salt
- 1 tbspn 70% dark chocolate chips
- ¼ teaspn lemon zest, grated finely

Directions

- Preheat now a mini waffle iron and then grease it.
- Place all Ingredients except chocolate chips and lemon zest and beat until well combined in a bowl.
- Gently, fold in the chocolate chips and lemon zest.

- Place ¼ of the mixture into preheated waffle iron and cooking for about minutes or until golden brown.
- Repeat now with the remaining mixture.
- Serve warm.

Nutrition:

Calories 278, Fat 8.3, Fiber 4.3, Carbs 8.8, Protein 23.7

Almond Chocolate Chaffle

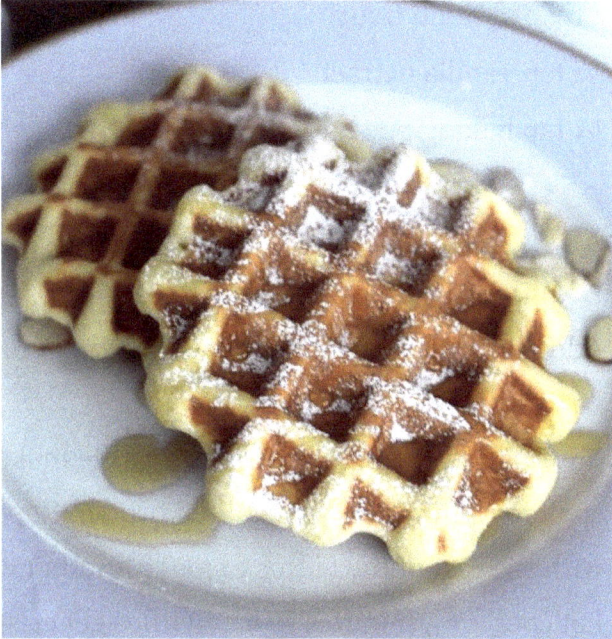

Preparation: 5 minutes

Cooking: 8 minutes

Servings: 2 chaffles

Ingredients

- 1 egg, beaten
- ½ cup of mozzarella cheese, shredded
- 2 tbsp almond chocolate chips, unsweetened

- 2 tbsp sweetener
- 1 tbsp whipping cream
- 1 tbsp almond flour
- ½ tsp vanilla extract
- ¼ tsp baking powder

Directions

1. Heat up your waffle maker.
2. Add all the chaffles Ingredients to a tiny mixing bowl and mix well.
3. Pour half of the batter into your waffle maker and cook for 4 minutes until golden brown. Repeat now with the rest of the batter to make another chaffle.
4. Let cool for 3 minutes to let chaffles get crispy.
5. Serve with blackberries, sweetener and enjoy!

Pumpkin Keto Protein Pumpkin Vanilla

Preparation: 30 minutes

Cooking: 10 minutes

Servings: 6

Ingredients

- 1 egg
- 1 tbspn of vanilla erithrite, passed through a sieve
- 1 pinch of cinnamon
- 15 grams of almond flour, passed through a sieve
- 1 teaspn of baking soda
- 120 grams of mozzarella, grated
- 50 grams of Hokkaido pumpkin, grated

Directions

1. Prepare the chaffle maker and switch it on so that it can Preheat now
2. In a tiny bowl, whisk the egg with the vanilla and cinnamon.
3. Gradually add baking soda and almond flour. I always sift it into the mix because I only work with

the whisk. The recipe is easy, and there is no need to get any dirty equipment.

4. Now add the mozzarella to the egg-flour mixture and stir with a fork until the cheese is well covered.
5. Finally, stir in the pumpkin.
6. Bake the chaffles in 2 portions over medium heat. The recipe makes 2 chaffles for my heart chaffle maker. The dough does not stick anywhere in me even without fat, even with lean mozzarella.
7. You should consume the finished chaffles immediately. For this reason, I make only half the recipe when my husband is not at home. You can't taste the cheese directly hot from the iron
8. When warming up in the microwave or the toaster, a slight taste of cheese reappears.
9. So maybe cut the recipe in half! Fresh tastes best.

Blueberries Syrup Chaffle

Preparation: 5 minutes

Cooking: 8 minutes

Servings: 2 chaffles

Ingredients

For chaffles:

- 1 egg, beaten
- ½ cup cheddar cheese, shredded
- 1 tsp almond flour
- 1 tsp sour cream
- A pinch of salt

For blueberries syrup:

- 1 cup fresh blueberries
- 1 tsp vanilla extract
- ¼ cup sweetener
- ¼ cup water

Directions

For blueberries syrup:

1. A saucepan over low heat adds the blueberries, water, sweetener, and vanilla extract.
2. Stir from time to time until you get a syrup.
3. Remove now from heat, set aside and let cool.

For chaffles:

4. Heat up your waffle maker.
5. Add all the chaffles Ingredients to a tiny mixing bowl and stir until well combined.
6. Pour half of the batter into your waffle maker and cook for 4 minutes until golden brown. Repeat now with the rest of the batter to make another chaffle.
7. Let cool for 3 minutes to let chaffles get crispy.
8. Top the chaffle with blueberries syrup.
9. Serve and enjoy!

Raspberry Mousse Chaffle

Preparation: 5 minutes

Cooking: 8 minutes

Servings: 2 chaffles

Ingredients

For chaffles:

- 1 large egg, beaten
- ½ cup mozzarella cheese, grated
- 1 tsp coconut flour
- 1 tsp water
- ¼ tsp baking powder

For mousse:

- 2 tbsp heavy whipping cream
- 2-3 tbsp fresh raspberries
- ½ tsp lemon zest
- ½ tsp vanilla extract
- 1-2 fresh mint leaves, for garnish

Directions

For mousse:

1. In a bowl, whip all the mousse Ingredients until fluffy. Set aside.

For chaffles:

- Heat up the mini waffle maker.
2. Add all the chaffles Ingredients to a tiny mixing bowl and combine well.
3. Pour half of the batter into your waffle maker and cook for 4 minutes until brown. Repeat now with the rest of the batter to make another chaffle.
4. Let cool for 3 minutes to let chaffles get crispy.
5. Top the chaffle with raspberry mousse and garnish with a fresh mint leaf.
6. Serve and enjoy!

Blackberries Syrup Chaffle

Preparation: 5 minutes

Cooking: 8 minutes

Servings: 2 chaffles

Ingredients

For chaffles:

- 1 egg, beaten
- ½ cup cheddar cheese, shredded
- 1 tsp almond flour
- 1 tsp sour cream
- A pinch of salt

For blackberries syrup:

- 1 cup fresh blackberries
- 1 tsp vanilla extract
- ¼ cup sweetener
- ¼ cup water

Directions

For blackberries syrup:

1. In a saucepan over low heat add the blackberries, water, sweetener, and vanilla extract.
2. Stir from time to time until you get a syrup.
3. Remove now from heat, set aside and let cool.

For chaffles:

4. Heat up your waffle maker.
5. Add all the chaffles Ingredients to a tiny mixing bowl and stir until well combined.
6. Pour half of the batter into your waffle maker and cook for 4 minutes until golden brown. Repeat now with the rest of the batter to make another chaffle.
7. Let cool for 3 minutes to let chaffles get crispy.
8. Top the chaffles with blackberries syrup.
9. Serve and enjoy!

Blackberry Cheesy Chaffle

Preparation: 5 minutes

Cooking: 20 minutes

Servings: 4 chaffles

Ingredients

For chaffles:

- 2 eggs, beaten
- 1 cup mozzarella cheese, shredded
- A pinch of salt

For topping:

- 1 ½ cup blackberries, minced
- 1 tsp lemon zest
- 2 tbsp lemon juice
- 1 tbsp sweetener
- 4 slices Brie cheese

Directions

For topping:

1. In a tiny saucepan over low heat, add blackberries, lemon zest, lemon juice and sweetener.

2. Cook for approx. 5 minutes until the sauce thickens. Remove now from heat and set aside.

For Chaffle:

1. Heat up your waffle maker and Preheat now oven at 400°.
2. Add all the chaffles Ingredients to a tiny mixing bowl and stir until well combined.
3. Pour ¼ of the batter into your waffle maker and cook for 4 minutes until golden brown. Repeat now with the rest of the batter to prepare the other chaffles.
4. Top the chaffle with brie and sauce.
5. Place the chaffles in a baking sheet lined with parchment paper and cook for 4-5 minutes until cheese bubbles.
6. Serve and enjoy!

Lemon Curd Chaffle

Preparation: 5 minutes

Cooking: 5 Minutes

Servings: 1

Ingredients

- 3 large eggs
- 4 oz. cream cheese, softened
- 1 Tbsp. low carb sweetener
- 1 tsp. vanilla extract
- ¾ cup Mozzarella cheese, shredded
- 3 Tbsp. coconut flour
- 1 tsp. baking powder
- ⅓ tsp. salt

For the lemon curd:

- ½-1 cup water
- 5 egg yolks
- ½ cup lemon juice
- ½ cup powdered sweetener
- 2 Tbsp. fresh lemon zest
- 1 tsp. vanilla extract

- Pinch of salt
- 8 Tbsp. cold butter, cubed

Directions

1. Pour water into a saucepan and heat over medium until it reaches a soft boil. Start with ½ cup and add more if needed.
2. Whisk yolks, lemon juice, lemon zest, powdered sweetener, vanilla, and salt in a medium heat-proof bowl. Leave to set for 5-6 minutes.
3. Place bowl onto saucepan and heat. The bowl shouldn't be touching water.
4. Whisk mixture for 8-10 min, or until it begins to thicken.
5. Add butter cubes and whisk for 7 min, until it thickens.
6. When it lightly coats the back of a spoon, Remove now from heat.
7. Refrigerate until cool, allowing it to continue thickening.
8. Turn on waffle maker to heat and oil it with cooking spray.
9. Add baking powder, coconut flour, and salt in a tiny bowl. Mix well and set aside.

10. Add eggs, cream cheese, sweetener, and vanilla in a separate bowl. Using a hand beater, beat until frothy.
11. Add Mozzarella to egg mixture and beat again.
12. Add dry Ingredients and Mix well until well-combined.
13. Add batter to waffle maker and cooking for 3-4 minutes.
14. Transfer to a plate and top with lemon curd before serving.

Nutrition:

Calories 579, Fat 18g, Carbs 33g, Protein 11 g

Walnut & Pumpkin Chaffles

Preparation: 5 minutes

Cooking: 10 Minutes

Servings: 2

Ingredients

- 1 organic egg, beaten
- ½ cup Mozzarella cheese, shredded
- 2 tbsps almond flour
- 1 tbspn sugar-free pumpkin puree
- 1 teaspn Erythritol
- ¼ teaspn ground cinnamon
- 2 tbsps walnuts, toasted and chopped

Directions

- Preheat now a mini waffle iron and then grease it.
- Place all Ingredients except walnuts and beat until well combined in a bowl.
- Fold in the walnuts.
- Place half of the mixture into preheated waffle iron and cooking for about 5 minutes or until golden brown.

- Repeat now with the remaining mixture.
- Serve warm.

Nutrition:

Calories 226, Fat 14g, Carbs 14g, Protein 8 g

Protein Rich Mozzarella Chaffles

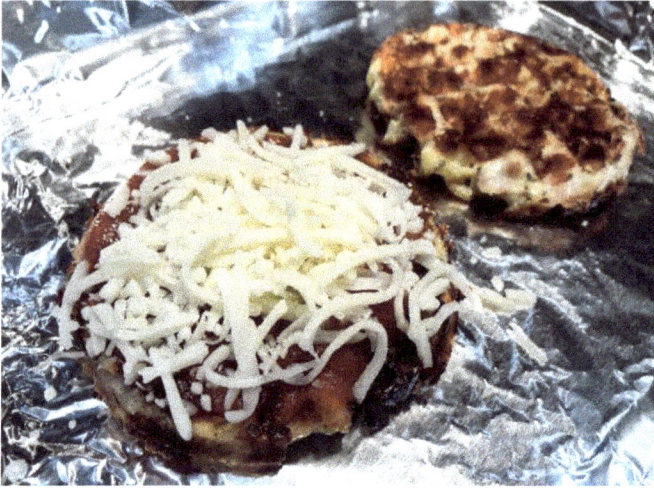

Preparation: 8 minutes

Cooking: 20 Minutes

Servings: 2

Ingredients

- ½ scoop unsweetened protein powder
- 2 large organic eggs
- ½ cup Mozzarella cheese, shredded
- 1 tbspn Erythritol
- ¼ teaspn organic vanilla extract

Directions

- Preheat now a mini waffle iron and then grease it.
- In a bowl, place all Ingredients and with a fork, Mix well until well combined.
- Place ¼ of the mixture into Preheated waffle iron and cooking for about 4-5 minutes or until golden brown.
- Repeat now with the remaining mixture.
- Serve warm.

Nutrition:

Calories 216, Fat 10g, Carbs 13g, Protein 10 g

Chocolate Chips Butter Chaffles

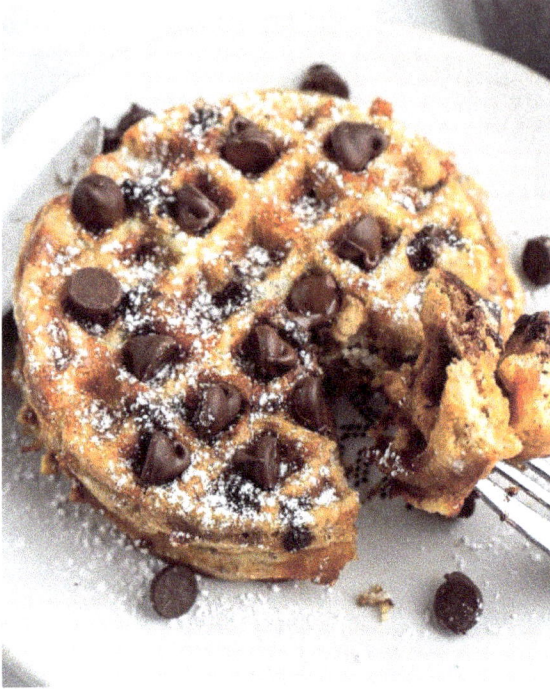

Preparation: 5 minutes

Cooking: 8 Minutes

Servings: 4

Ingredients

- 1 organic egg, beaten
- ¼ cup Mozzarella cheese, shredded

- 2 tbsps creamy peanut butter
- 1 tbspn almond flour
- 1 tbspn granulated Erythritol
- 1 teaspn organic vanilla extract
- 1 tbspn 70% dark chocolate chips

Directions
- Preheat now a mini waffle iron and then grease it.
- Place all Ingredients except chocolate chips and beat until well combined in a bowl.
- Gently, fold in the chocolate chips.
- Place half of the mixture into Preheated waffle iron and cooking for about minutes or until golden brown.
- Repeat now with the remaining mixture.
- Serve warm.

Nutrition:

Calories 336, Fat 22g, Carbs 12g, Protein 18g

Pumpkin Chaffles

Preparation: 5 minutes

Cooking: 12 Minutes

Servings: 3

Ingredients

- 1 organic egg, beaten
- ½ cup Mozzarella cheese, shredded
- 1½ tbspn homemade pumpkin puree
- ½ teaspn Erythritol
- ½ teaspn organic vanilla extract
- ¼ teaspn pumpkin pie spice

Directions

1. Preheat now a mini waffle iron and then grease it.
2. In a bowl, place all the Ingredients and beat until well combined.
3. Place ¼ of the mixture into Preheated waffle iron and cooking for about 4-6 minutes or until golden brown.
4. Repeat now with the remaining mixture.

5. Serve warm.

Nutrition:

Calories 316, Fat 2g, Carbs 10g, Protein 18g

Shredded Mozzarella Chaffles

Preparation: 5 minutes

Cooking: 8 Minutes

Servings: 2

Ingredients

- 1 large organic egg
- 1 teaspn coconut flour
- 1 teaspn Erythritol
- ½ teaspn organic vanilla extract
- ½ cup Mozzarella cheese, shredded finely
- 2 tbsps 70% dark chocolatc chips

Directions

- Preheat now a mini waffle iron and then grease it.
- In a bowl, place the egg, coconut flour, sweetener and vanilla extract and beat until well combined.
- Add the cheese and stir to combine.
- Place half of the mixture into Preheated waffle iron and top with half of the chocolate chips.
- Place a little egg mixture over each chocolate chip.

- Cooking for about 3-4 minutes or until golden brown.
- Repeat now with the remaining mixture and chocolate chips.
- Serve warm.

Nutrition:

Calories 247, Fat 6g, Carbs 13g, Protein 21 g

Cream Cake Chaffle

Preparation: 8 minutes

Cooking: 12 Minutes

Servings: 2

Ingredients

Chaffle:

- 4 oz. cream cheese, softened
- 4 eggs
- 4 tbsp. coconut flour
- 1 tbsp. almond flour
- 1 ½ tsp. baking powder
- 1 tbsp. butter, softened
- 1 tsp. vanilla extract
- ½ tsp. cinnamon
- 1 tbsp. sweetener
- 1 tbsp. shredded coconut, colored and unsweetened
- 1 tbsp. walnuts, chopped

Italian Cream Frosting:

- 2 oz. cream cheese, softened

- 2 tbsp. butter, room temperature
- 2 tbsp. sweetener
- ½ tsp. vanilla

Directions

1. Preheat now your waffle maker and add ¼ of the
2. Cooking for 3 minutes and repeat the process until you have 4 chaffles.
3. Remove now and set aside.
4. In the meantime, start making your frosting by mixing all the
5. Stir until you have a smooth and creamy mixture.
6. Cool, frost the cake and enjoy.

Nutrition:

Calories 231, Fat 16g, Carbs 13g, Protein 28g

2 Layered Chaffles

Preparation: 5 minutes

Cooking: 10 Minutes

Servings: 2

Ingredients

- 1 organic egg, beaten and divided
- ½ cup cheddar cheese, shredded and divided
- Pinch of salt

Directions

1. Preheat now a mini waffle iron and then grease it.
2. Place about 1/8 cup of cheese in the bottom of the waffle iron and top with half of the beaten egg.
3. Now, place 1/8 cup of cheese on top and cooking for about 4–5 minutes.
4. Repeat now with the remaining cheese and egg.
5. Serve warm.

Nutrition:

Calories 106, Fat 26g, Carbs 8g, Protein 32 g

Cream Mini-Chaffle

Preparation: 5 minutes

Cooking: 10 Minutes

Servings: 2

Ingredients

- 2 tsp. coconut flour
- 4 tsp. swerve/monk fruit
- ¼ tsp. baking powder
- 1 egg
- 1 oz. cream cheese
- ½ tsp. vanilla extract

Directions

1. Turn on waffle maker to heat and oil it with cooking spray.
2. Mix swerve/monk fruit, coconut flour, and baking powder in a tiny mixing bowl.
3. Add cream cheese, egg, vanilla extract, and whisk until well-combined.
4. Add batter into waffle maker and cooking for 3-min, until golden brown.

5. Serve with your favorite toppings.

Nutrition:

Calories: 210, Fat: 9g, Carbohydrates: 10.9g

Raspberries Chaffles

Preparation: 5 minutes

Cooking: 5 Minutes

Servings: 5

Ingredients

- 4 Tbsp. almond flour
- 4 large eggs
- 2⅓ cup shredded Mozzarella cheese
- 1 tsp. vanilla extract
- 1 Tbsp. erythritol sweetener
- 1½ tsp. baking powder
- ½ cup raspberries

Directions

1. Turn on waffle maker to heat and oil it with cooking spray.
2. Mix almond flour, sweetener, and baking powder in a bowl.
3. Add cheese, eggs, and vanilla extract, and Mix well until well-combined.

4. Add 1 portion of batter to waffle maker and spread it evenly. Close and cooking for 3-min, or until golden.
5. Repeat until remaining batter is used.
6. Serve with raspberries.

Nutrition:

Calories: 338, Fat: 14g, Carbohydrates: 5.9g

Keto Snicker Chaffle

Preparation: 5 minutes

Cooking: 10 minutes

Servings: 2

Ingredients

- 1 Egg
- 1/2 cup Mozzarella Cheese
- 2 tbsp Almond Flour
- 1 tbsp Lakanto Golden Sweetener
- 1/2 tsp Vanilla Extract
- 1/4 tsp Cinnamon
- 1/2 tsp Baking Powder
- 1/4 tsp Cream of tartar, optional

Coating:

- 1 tbsp Butter
- 2 tbsp Lakanto Classic Sweetener
- 1/2 tsp Cinnamon

Directions

1. Preheat now your mini waffle maker.
2. In a tiny bowl, combine all chaffle Ingredients.
3. Pour half of the chaffle mixture onto the waffle iron center. Allow to cooke for 3-5 minutes.
4. Carefully remove now and repeat for second chaffle. Allow chaffles to cool so that they crisp.
5. In a tiny bowl, combine sweetener and cinnamon for coating.
6. Melt now butter in a tiny microwave safe bowl and brush the chaffles with the butter.
7. Sprinkle sweetener and cinnamon mixture on both sides of the chaffles once they1re brushed with butter.

Nutrition:

Calories: 182, Total Fat: 13.75g, Carbohydrates: 2g, Net Carbohydrates: 1.5g, Fiber: 0.5g, Protein: 11.5g

Keto Chaffle Churro

Preparation: 10 minutes

Cooking: 6-10 minutes | **Servings:** 1

Ingredients

- 1 Egg
- 1 Tbsp. Almond flour
- ½ tsp. Vanilla extract
- 1 tsp. Cinnamon divided
- ¼ tsp. Baking powder
- ½ C. Shredded mozzarella
- 1 Tbsp. Swerve confectioners sugar substitute
- 1 Tbsp. Swerve brown sugar substitute
- 1 Tbsp. Butter Melted

Directions

1. Preheat now your mini waffle maker.
2. Add the egg, almond flour, vanilla extract, ½ tsp of cinnamon, baking powder, shredded mozzarella and the Swerve confectioners sugar substitute into a bowl, and mix to combine well.

3. Place an even layer of half of the mixture into the mini waffle maker, and cook for 3-5 min, or until your desired level of doneness has been reached. A longer cook time will give you a crispier chaffle.

4. Remove now the first chaffle from the mini waffle maker, and place the second half of the batter into it. Cook the second chaffle for 3-5 minutes.

5. Cut the two chaffles into strips.

6. Place the cut strips into a bowl and cover in the melted butter.

7. Mix now the Swerve brown sugar substitute and the remaining ½ tsp of cinnamon in a bowl to combine well.

8. Pour the cinnamon sugar mixture over the churro chaffle strips in the mixing bowl, and toss to coat them well.

Keto Chaffle Cheddar

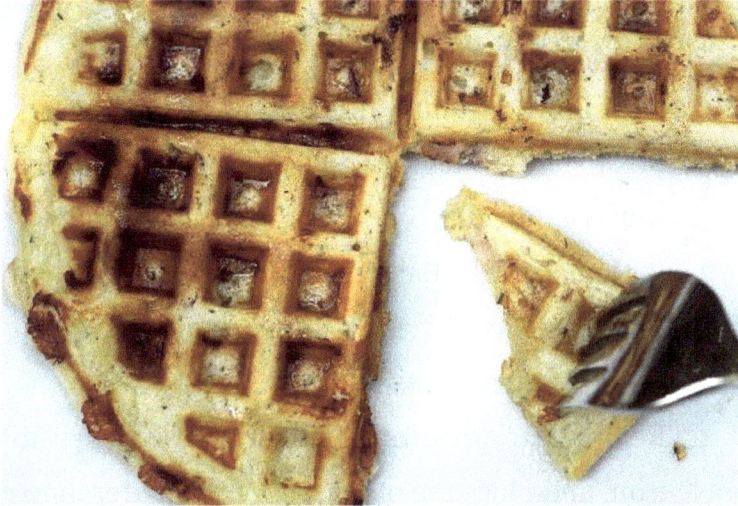

Preparation: 5 minutes+

Cooking: 3-5 minutes

Servings: 1

Ingredients

- 1 Egg
- ⅓ Cup Shredded cheddar cheese
- 1 ½ Tbsp. Heavy whipping cream
- 1 Tbsp. Almond flour
- Salt and pepper to taste

- Mini waffle iron

Directions

1. Heat up your mini waffle iron.
2. Mix together the Ingredients in a mixing bowl until well combined.
3. Place half of the batter mixture into the mini waffle maker, and cook for 3-5 min, or until the chaffle is done to your liking.
4. Remove now the first chaffle from the mini waffle iron, and place the other half of the batter in to cook.

Keto Chaffles Caramel

Preparation: 10 minutes+

Cooking: 15 minutes

Servings: 2

Ingredients

For the chaffles:

- 1 Tbsp. Swerve confectioners sugar substitute
- 2 Tbsp. Almond flour
- 1 Egg
- ½ tsp. Vanilla extract
- ⅓ C. Shredded mozzarella cheese

For the caramel sauce:

- 3 Tbsp. Butter unsalted
- 2 Tbsp. Swerve brown sugar substitute
- ⅓ C. Heavy whipping cream
- ½ tsp. Vanilla extract

Directions

1. Preheat now your mini waffle maker.

2. Place the 3 tbsps of butter and the 2 tbsps of brown sugar substitute together in a tiny skillet or pan over medium heat on the stove.
3. Cook the butter and sugar substitute mixture for 4-5 minutes until it begins to brown but not burn.
4. Add the heavy whipping cream into the mixture on the stove, and whisk it in well. Cook the mixture on a low boil for 10 minutes until the mixture thickens and has the color of caramel sauce.
5. While the caramel sauce is cooking, mix now the Ingredients for the chaffles in a mixing bowl.
6. Place half of the chaffle mixture into the heated mini waffle maker, and cook for 3-5 minutes until your desired level of doneness has been reached.
7. Remove now the first chaffle, and cook the second half of the batter for another 3-5 minutes.
8. Take the finished caramel sauce off the heat, and add in the vanilla extract. Let cool slightly.
9. Pour the caramel sauce over the chaffles and serve.

Chocolate Chip Vanilla Chaffles

Preparation: 1 minute +

Cooking: 4 minutes

Servings: 2

Ingredients

- 1/2 cup pre-shredded/grated mozzarella
- 1 egg
- 1 tbsp granulated sweetener of choice or more to your taste
- 1 tsp vanilla extract
- 2 tbsp almond meal/flour
- 1 tbsp sugar-free chocolate chips or cacao nibs

Directions

1. Combine the Ingredients in a bowl.
2. Preheat now the mini waffle maker. When it is hot spray with olive oil and pour half the batter into your waffle maker.
3. Cook for 2-4 minutes then remove and repeat.

4. Top, serve, and enjoy.

Nutrition:

Fat 28.1g 43%, Sodium 562mg 24%, Potassium 171mg 5%, Total Carbohydrates 8.2g 3%, Fiber 1.8g 8%, Sugar 1.6g 2%, Protein 24.7g 49%

Pumpkin and Psyllium Husk Chaffles

Preparation: 8 minutes

Cooking: 16 Minutes

Servings: 2

Ingredients

- 2 organic eggs
- ½ cup Mozzarella cheese, shredded
- 1 tbspn homemade pumpkin puree
- 2 teaspns Erythritol
- ½ teaspn psyllium husk powder
- 1/3 teaspn ground cinnamon
- Pinch of salt
- ½ teaspn organic vanilla extract

Directions

1. Preheat now a mini waffle iron and then grease it.
2. In a bowl, place all Ingredients and beat until well combined.

3. Place ¼ of the mixture into preheated waffle iron and cooking for about 4 minutes or until golden brown.
4. Repeat now with the remaining mixture.
5. Serve warm.

Nutrition:

Calories: 332, Fat: 15.5g, Carbohydrates: 17.1g, Protein: 27.7g

Chicken Chaffles With Tzatziki

Preparation: 6 minutes

Cooking: 12 Minutes

Servings: 2

Ingredients

Chaffles:

- 1 organic egg, beaten
- 1/3 cup of grass-fed cooked chicken, chopped 1/3 cup of Mozzarella cheese, shredded
- ¼ teaspn garlic, minced
- ¼ teaspn dried basil, crushed

Tzatziki:

- ¼ cup plain Greek yogurt
- ½ of tiny cucumber, peeled, seeded, and chopped
- 1 teaspn olive oil
- ½ teaspn fresh lemon juice
- Pinch of ground black pepper
- ¼ tbspn fresh dill, chopped
- ½ of garlic clove, peeled

Directions

1. Preheat now a mini waffle iron and then grease it.
2. For chaffles: In a bowl, put all Ingredients and mix well until well combined with your hands. Place half of the mixture into preheated waffle iron and cooking for about 4-6 minutes.
3. Repeat now with the remaining mixture.
4. Meanwhile, in a food processor, for tzatziki, place all the Ingredients and pulse until well combined.
5. Serve warm chaffles alongside the tzatziki.

Nutrition:

Calories 338, Fat 3g, Carbs 23g, Protein 21 g

Banana Chaffle

Preparation: 5 minutes

Cooking: 4 minutes

Servings: 1 chaffle

Ingredients

- 1 tbsp heavy whipping cream
- 1 tbsp sweetener
- 1 tbsp coconut flour
- 1 egg
- ½ cup mozzarella cheese, shredded
- ½ tsp vanilla extract
- 1 tsp banana extract
- 1 tbsp nuts, chopped

Directions

1. Heat up your waffle maker.
2. Add all the Ingredients to a tiny mixing bowl and mix well.

3. Pour the batter into your waffle maker and cook for 4 minutes until golden brown.
4. Let cool for 3 minutes to let chaffle get crispy.
5. Serve with sugar free maple syrup and enjoy!

Creamy Chaffle

Preparation: 5 minutes

Cooking: 16 minutes

Servings: 4 chaffles

Ingredients

For chaffles:

- 2 tbsp cream cheese
- 2 eggs
- 1 cup mozzarella cheese, shredded
- 1 tbsp butter, Melted
- 1 tsp vanilla extract
- ½ tsp cinnamon
- 1 tbsp sweetener
- 1 tbsp coconut flour
- 1 tbsp almond flour
- 1 tsp baking powder
- 1 tbs chopped walnuts

Ingredients for cream:

- 4 tbsp cream cheese

- 2 tbsp butter
- 2 tsp sweetener
- ½ tsp vanilla

Directions

1. Heat up your waffle maker.
2. Add in a blender all the Ingredients for the chaffles and blend until creamy.
3. Pour ¼ of the batter into your waffle maker and cook for 4 minutes. Repeat now with the rest of the batter to make the other chaffles.
4. Let cool for 3 minutes to let chaffles get crispy.
5. A tiny mixing bowl adds all the Ingredients for the cream and stir them till smoothy.
6. Frost the cooled chaffles with the cream.
7. Serve and enjoy!

Peanut Butter Creamy Chaffle

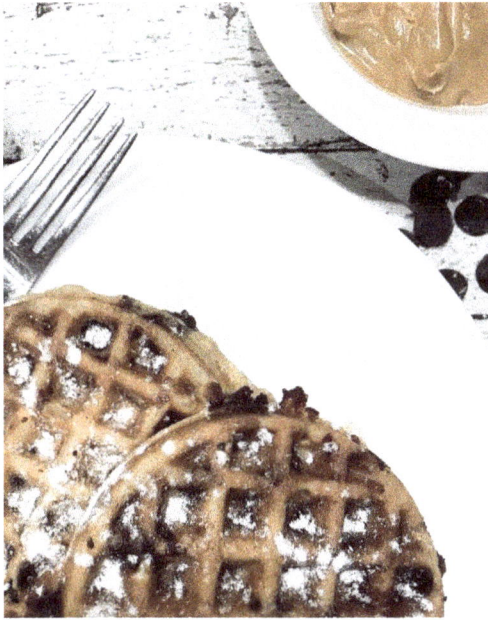

Preparation: 5 minutes

Cooking: 8 minutes

Servings: 2 chaffles

Ingredients

For chaffles:

- 1 large egg, beaten
- ½ cup shredded mozzarella cheese

- 1 tbsp almond flour
- ½ tsp baking powder

For peanut butter cream:

- 2 tbsp keto peanut butter
- 1 tsp sweetener
- 1 tbsp heavy cream

Directions

For peanut butter cream:

1. Blend all Ingredients in a tiny bowl. Set aside.

For chaffles:

1. Heat up your waffle maker.
2. Add all the chaffles Ingredients to a tiny mixing bowl and stir until well combined.
3. Pour half of the batter into your waffle maker and cook for 4 minutes until golden brown. Repeat now with the rest of the batter to make another chaffle.
4. Spread the chaffles with peanut butter cream.
5. Serve and enjoy!

Chaffle & Custard

Preparation: 5 minutes

Cooking: 15 minutes

Servings: 2 chaffles

Ingredients

For chaffles:

- 1 tbsp almond flour
- ½ cup mozzarella cheese
- 1 egg, beaten
- 1 tbsp sweetener
- ½ tsp vanilla extract

For custard:

- 2 eggs
- 2 tbsp heavy cream
- 1 tbsp brown sugar substitute
- ½ tsp cinnamon powder
- ½ tsp vanilla extract

Directions

<u>For custard:</u>

1. Preheat now the oven at 350 °.
2. Place all Ingredients in a tiny bowl and stir until well combined.
3. Pour the mixture in a baking tin and bake it for about 40-45 minutes.
4. Remove now from heat and set aside to cool.

<u>For chaffles:</u>

1. Heat up your waffle maker.
2. Add all the chaffles Ingredients to a tiny mixing bowl and combine well.
3. Pour ½ of the batter into your waffle maker and cook for 4 minutes until golden brown. Then cook the remaining batter to make another chaffle.
4. Top the chaffles with custard.
5. Serve and enjoy!

Raspberry & Custard Chaffle

Preparation: 5 minutes

Cooking: 55 minutes

Servings: 2 chaffles

Ingredients

For chaffles:

- 1 tbsp almond flour
- ½ cup mozzarella cheese
- 1 egg, beaten
- 1 tbsp sweetener
- ½ tsp vanilla extract

For custard:

- 2 eggs
- 2 tbsp heavy cream
- 1 tbsp brown sugar substitute
- ½ tsp cinnamon powder
- ½ tsp vanilla extract

For topping:

- 2 tbsp of fresh raspberries

Directions

<u>For custard:</u>

1. Preheat now the oven at 350 °.
2. Place all Ingredients in a tiny bowl and stir until well combined.
3. Pour the mixture in a baking tin and bake it for about 40-45 minutes.
4. Remove now from heat and set aside to cool.

<u>For chaffles:</u>

1. Heat up your waffle maker.
2. Add all the chaffles Ingredients to a tiny mixing bowl and combine well.
3. Pour ½ of the batter into your waffle maker and cook for 4 minutes until golden brown. Then cook the remaining batter to make another chaffle.
4. Top the chaffles with custard and sprinkle with raspberries.
5. Serve and enjoy!

Yogurt Chaffle & Blueberries

Preparation: 5 minutes

Cooking: 8 minutes

Servings: 2 chaffles

Ingredients

- ½ cup mozzarella cheese, shredded
- 1 egg, beaten
- 1 tbsp yogurt
- 1 tbsp fresh blueberries, chopped
- ¼ tsp baking powder

Directions

1. Heat up the mini waffle maker.
2. Add all the Ingredients to a tiny mixing bowl and stir until well combined.
3. Pour half of the batter into your waffle maker and cook for 4 minutes until brown. Repeat now with the rest of the batter to prepare another chaffle.
4. Serve and enjoy!

Strawberry Yogurt Chaffle

Preparation: 5 minutes

Cooking: 8 minutes

Servings: 2 chaffles

Ingredients

- ½ cup mozzarella cheese, shredded
- 1 egg, beaten
- 1 tbsp yogurt
- 1 tbsp fresh strawberries, chopped
- ¼ tsp baking powder

Directions

1. Heat up your waffle maker.
2. Add all the Ingredients to a tiny mixing bowl and stir until well combined.
3. Pour half of the batter into your waffle maker and cook for 4 minutes until brown. Repeat now with the rest of the batter to prepare another chaffle.
4. Serve and enjoy!

Vanilla Chaffle with Lemon Icing

Preparation: 5 minutes

Cooking: 8 minutes

Servings: 2 chaffles

Ingredients

For chaffles:

- 1 tbsp almond flour
- ½ cup mozzarella cheese
- 1 egg, beaten
- 1 tbsp sweetener
- ½ tsp vanilla extract

For lemon icing:

- 2 tbsp powdered erythritol
- 4 tsp heavy cream
- 1 tsp lemon juice
- Lemon zest

Directions

1. Heat up your waffle maker.

2. Add all the Ingredients for the chaffles to a tiny mixing bowl and combine well.
3. Pour ½ of the batter into your waffle maker and cook for 4 minutes. Then cook the remaining batter to make another chaffle.
4. Combine in a mixing bowl the powdered erythritol, heavy cream, lemon juice and lemon
5. zest.
6. Pour over vanilla chaffle. Serve and enjoy!

White Chocolate Chaffle with Glaze and Raspberries

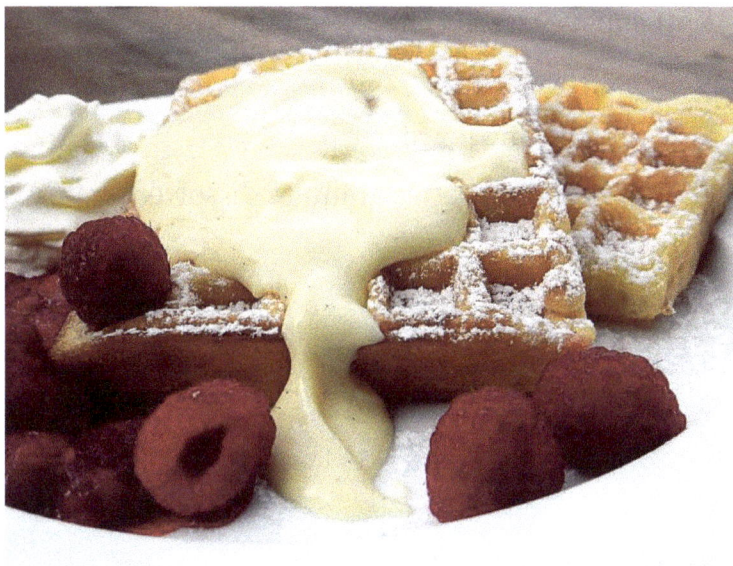

Preparation: 5 minutes

Cooking: 16 minutes

Servings: 4 chaffles

Ingredients

For chaffles:

- 2 eggs, beaten

- 1 tbsp butter, Melted
- 1 tbsp softened cream cheese
- 2 tbsp unsweetened white chocolate chips
- 1 cup mozzarella cheese, shredded
- 2 tbsp sweetener
- ½ tsp baking powder
- ½ tsp instant coffee granules dissolved in 1 tbspn hot water
- ½ tsp vanilla extract
- A pinch of salt

For glaze:

- 1 egg yolk
- ¼ cup heavy cream
- 2 tbsp sweetener
- 1 tbsp butter
- ½ tsp caramel
- ¼ cup pecans, chopped
- ¼ cup unsweetened flaked coconut
- 1 tsp coconut flour
- 2 tbsp of fresh raspberries for topping

Directions

For chaffles:

1. Heat up the mini waffle maker.
2. Add all the chaffles Ingredients to a tiny mixing bowl and mix well.
3. Pour ¼ of the batter into your waffle maker and cook for 4 minutes. Repeat now with the rest of the batter to make 3 more chaffles.
4. Let cool for 3 minutes to let chaffles get crispy.

For glaze:

5. Combine the egg yolk, heavy cream, butter, and sweetener in a pan over medium heat.
6. Simmer slowly for approx. 4 minutes.
7. Remove now from heat and stir in extract, pecans, flaked coconut, and coconut flour.
8. Top the chaffle with the glaze and the raspberries.
9. Serve and enjoy!

New Year Chaffle With Coconut Cream

Preparation: 7 minutes

Cooking: 5 minutes

Servings: 2

Ingredients:

- 2 large eggs
- 1/8 cup almond flour
- 1 tsp. cinnamon powder
- 1 tsp. sea salt
- 1/2 tsp. baking soda
- 1 cup shredded Mozzarella

For Topping:

- 2 tbsps. coconut cream
- 1 tbsp. unsweetened chocolate sauce

Directions

1. Preheat now waffle maker according to the manufacturer's directions.
2. Mix recipe Ingredients in a mixing bowl.
3. Add cheese and mix well.

4. Pour about ½ cup mixture into your waffle maker's center and cook for about 2-3 minute until golden and crispy.
5. Repeat now with the remaining batter.
6. For serving, coat coconut cream over chaffles. Drizzle chocolate sauce over chaffle.
7. Freeze chaffle in the freezer for about 10 minutes
8. Serve on Christmas morning and enjoy!

Nutrition:

Kcal 225, Fat 17.4g, Net Carbs 2g, Protein 15g

Chaffles And Ice-cream Platter

Preparation: 7 minutes

Cooking: 5 minutes

Ingredients

- 2 keto brownie chaffles
- 2 scoop vanilla keto ice cream
- 8 oz. strawberries, sliced
- keto chocolate sauce

Directions

1. Arrange chaffles, ice-cream, strawberries slice in serving plate.
2. Drizzle chocolate sauce on top.
3. Serve and enjoy!

Nutrition:

Kcal 345, Fat 12g, Net Carbs 4g, Protein 24g

Choco Chip Pumpkin Chaffle

Preparation: 20 minutes

Cooking: 15 Minutes

Servings: 2

Ingredients

- 1 egg, lightly beaten
- 1 tbsp. almond flour
- 1 tbsp. unsweetened chocolate chips
- 1/4 tsp. pumpkin pie spice
- 2 tbsp. Swerve
- 1 tbsp. pumpkin puree
- 1/2 cup Mozzarella cheese, shredded

Directions

1. Preheat now your waffle maker.
2. In a tiny bowl, mix egg and pumpkin puree.
3. Add pumpkin pie spice, Swerve, almond flour, and cheese and mix well.
4. Stir in chocolate chips.

5. Spray waffle maker with cooking spray.
6. Pour half batter in the hot waffle maker and cooking for 4 minutes. Repeat now with the remaining batter.
7. Serve and enjoy.

Nutrition:

Kcal: 453, Fat: 31g, Net Carbs: 6g, Protein: 43g

Chocolate Creamy Chaffle

Preparation: 5 minutes

Cooking: 16 minutes

Servings: 4 chaffles

Ingredients

For chaffles:

- 2 tbsp cream cheese
- 2 eggs
- 1 cup mozzarella cheese, shredded
- 1 tbsp butter, Melted
- 1 tsp vanilla extract
- 1 tbsp sweetener
- 1 tbsp coconut flour
- 1 tbsp almond flour
- 1 tsp baking powder
- 2 tbsp chocolate chips, unsweetened

For cream:

- 4 tbsp cream cheese
- 2 tbsp butter

- 2 tsp sweetener
- ½ tsp vanilla

Directions

1. Heat up your waffle maker.
2. Add to a blender all the Ingredients for the chaffles and blend until creamy.
3. Pour ¼ of the batter into your waffle maker and cook for 4 minutes. Repeat now with the rest of the batter to make the other chaffles.
4. Let cool for 3 minutes to let chaffles get crispy.
5. A tiny mixing bowl adds all the Ingredients for the cream and stir them till smoothy.
6. Frost the chaffles with the cream.
7. Serve and enjoy!

Chaffle with Jicama

Preparation: 5 minutes

Cooking: 45 minutes

Servings: 5 chaffles

Ingredients

For the filling:

- 2 cups jicama, diced
- ¼ cup sweetener
- 4 tbsp butter
- 1 tsp cinnamon
- 1/8 tsp nutmeg
- ¼ tsp cloves, ground
- ½ tsp vanilla extract
- 20 drops apple flavoring

For the chaffles:

- 2 eggs
- 1 cup mozzarella cheese, grated
- 1 tbsp almond flour
- 1 tsp coconut flour

- ½ tsp baking powder

For the icing:

- 1 tbsp butter
- 2 tsp heavy cream
- 3 tbsp powdered sweetener
- ¼ tsp vanilla extract

Directions

For the filling:

1. In a saucepan over medium heat, add melted butter, sweetener, and jicama.
2. Simmer approx. 20 minutes until the jicama is soft.
3. Remove now from heat and stir in the spices and flavorings.

For the chaffles:

4. Heat up your waffle maker.
5. Add all the Ingredients to a tiny mixing bowl and combine well. Stir the jicama mix into the egg batter.
6. Pour 1/5 of the batter into your waffle maker and cook for 4 minutes. Repeat now with the rest of the batter to make 4 more chaffles.
7. Let cool for 3 minutes to let chaffles get crispy.

Directions for the icing:

8. In a tiny pan add melted butter, sweetener, and heavy cream.
9. Simmer for 4-5 min, until thickened. Add vanilla.
10. Top the chaffles with jicama filling and put the hot glaze over the chaffles.
11. Serve and enjoy!

Chaffle with Chocolate Icing

Preparation: 5 minutes

Cooking: 8 minutes

Servings: 2 chaffles

Ingredients

For the chaffles:

- 2 eggs, beaten
- ½ cup mozzarella cheese, shredded
- ½ tsp baking powder
- 1 tsp vanilla extract
- 2 tbsp erythritol
- 3 tbsp almond milk

For the chocolate icing:

- ¼ cup powdered erythritol
- 1 tbsp cocoa powder
- 1 tbsp almond milk
- ½ tsp vanilla extract

Directions

1. Heat up your waffle maker.
2. Add all the Ingredients for chaffles to a tiny mixing bowl. Stir until well combined.
3. Pour half of the batter into your waffle maker and cook for 4 minutes. Repeat now with the rest of the batter to make another chaffle.
4. Let cool for 3 minutes to let chaffles get crispy.
5. Add all the Ingredients for the chocolate glaze to a tiny bowl and combine well.
6. Top each chaffle with glaze.
7. Serve and enjoy!

White Chocolate Macadamia Syrup Chaffle

Preparation: 5 minutes

Cooking: 8 minutes

Servings: 2 chaffles

Ingredients

For chaffles:

- 1 egg
- ½ cup mozzarella cheese, grated
- 1 tsp coconut flour
- 1 tsp water
- ¼ tsp baking powder

For glaze:

- 2 tbsp white chocolate chips, unsweetened
- 1 cup of coconut milk
- 2 tsp macadamia nut syrup

Directions

<u>For glaze:</u>

1. In a saucepan, warm up the coconut milk. Remove now from heat and add white chocolate chips and macadamia nut syrup.
2. Wait 5 minutes before stirring. Set aside to allow mixture to cool.

<u>For chaffles:</u>

3. Heat up the mini waffle maker.
4. Add all the Ingredients to a tiny mixing bowl and combine well.
5. Pour half of the batter into your waffle maker and cook for 4 minutes until brown. Repeat now with the rest of the batter to make another chaffle.
6. Let cool for 3 minutes to let chaffles get crispy.
7. Serve each chaffle with chocolate glaze and enjoy!

Sweet Eggnog Chaffle

Preparation: 5 minutes

Cooking: 8 minutes

Servings: 2 chaffles

Ingredients

For chaffles:

- 1 egg, beaten
- 2 tbsp cream cheese, softened
- 2 tsp sweetener
- 2 tbsp coconut flour
- ½ tsp baking powder
- ¼ cup keto eggnog
- A pinch of nutmeg

For topping:

- 2 tbsp keto whipped cream
- 2 tbsp fresh blackberries
- 2 tsp lemon juice

Directions

1. Heat up your waffle maker.
2. Add all the chaffles Ingredients to a tiny mixing bowl and stir until well combined.
3. Pour half of the batter into your waffle maker and cook for 4 minutes until golden brown. Repeat now with the rest of the batter to make another chaffle.
4. Let cool for 3 minutes to let chaffles get crispy.
5. In a tiny bowl, combine the lemon juice and blackberries.
6. Spread the chaffle with whipped cream and top with blackberries.
7. Serve and enjoy!

Chaffle with Ricotta Cheese

Preparation: 5 minutes

Cooking: 16 minutes

Servings: 4 chaffles

Ingredients

For the chaffles:

- 1 egg
- 1 egg yolk
- 3 tbsp melted butter
- 1 tbsp swerve confectioner's sugar substitute
- 1 cup parmesan cheese, grated
- 2 tbsp mozzarella cheese, shredded

For the topping:

- ½ cup ricotta cheese
- 2 tbsp swerve confectioner's sugar substitute
- 1 tsp vanilla extract

Directions

<u>For the topping:</u>

1. In a tiny mixing bowl stir ricotta cheese, vanilla extract and swerve confectioner's sugar substitute until creamy.

<u>For chaffles:</u>

2. Heat up your waffle maker.
3. Add all the chaffles Ingredients in a tiny mixing bowl and stir until well combined.
4. Pour 1/4 of the batter into your waffle maker and cook for 4 minutes until brown. Repeat now with the rest of the batter to make the other chaffles.
5. Let cool for 3 minutes to let chaffles get crispy.
6. Top each chaffle with ricotta filling.
7. Serve and enjoy!

Ricotta and Chocolate Chaffle

Preparation: 5 minutes

Cooking: 16 minutes

Servings: 4 chaffles

Ingredients

For the chaffles:

- 1 egg
- 1 egg yolk
- 3 tbsp Melted butter
- 1 tbsp swerve confectioner's sugar substitute
- 1 cup parmesan cheese, grated
- 2 tbsp mozzarella cheese, shredded

For the topping:

- ½ cup ricotta cheese
- 2 tbsp swerve confectioner's sugar substitute
- 1 tsp vanilla extract
- 2 tbsp milk chocolate chips, unsweetened

Directions

<u>For the topping:</u>

1. In a tiny mixing bowl stir ricotta cheese, vanilla extract and swerve confectioner's sugar substitute until creamy.
2. Add the chocolate chips and mix well.

<u>For chaffles:</u>

3. Heat up your waffle maker.
4. Add all the chaffles Ingredients in a tiny mixing bowl and stir until well combined.
5. Pour ¼ of the batter into your waffle maker and cook for 4 minutes until brown. Repeat now with the rest of the batter to make the other chaffles.
6. Let cool for 3 minutes to let chaffles get crispy.
7. Top each chaffle with ricotta and chocolate filling.
8. Serve and enjoy!

Nuts and Ricotta Chaffles

Preparation: 5 minutes

Cooking: 16 minutes

Servings: 4 chaffles

Ingredients

For the chaffles:

- 1 egg
- 1 egg yolk
- 3 tbsp Melt nowed butter
- 1 tbsp swerve confectioner's sugar substitute
- 1 cup parmesan cheese, grated
- 2 tbsp mozzarella cheese, shredded

For the topping:

- ½ cup ricotta cheese
- 2 tbsp swerve confectioner's sugar substitute
- 1 tsp vanilla extract
- 2 tbsp nuts, minced

Directions

For the topping:

1. In a tiny mixing bowl stir ricotta cheese, vanilla extract and swerve confectioner's sugar substitute until creamy.
2. Add the minced nuts and mix well.

For chaffles:

1. Heat up your waffle maker.
2. Add all the chaffles Ingredients to a tiny mixing bowl and stir until well combined.
3. Pour ¼ of the batter into your waffle maker and cook for 4 minutes until brown. Repeat now with the rest of the batter to make the other chaffles.
4. Let cool for 3 minutes to let chaffles get crispy.
5. Top each chaffle with ricotta filling.
6. Serve and enjoy!

www.ingramcontent.com/pod-product-compliance
Lightning Source LLC
Chambersburg PA
CBHW050755030426
42336CB00012B/1831